International College of Integrative Manual Therapy™ Wellness Series

Ex 2: Functional Exercise Program for Head and Neck Problems

Manual Therapy for the Pelvis, Sacrum, Cervical, Thoracic and Lumbar Spine, with Muscle Energy Technique—A Contemporary Clinical Analysis of Biomechanics

Integrative Manual Therapy for the Autonomic Nervous System and Related Disorders

Integrative Manual Therapy for the Upper and Lower Extremities

Dialogues in Contemporary Rehabilitation for Prevention and Care

Ex1

Functional Exercise Program for Women's and Men's Health Issues

Developed by

Dr. Sharon (Weiselfish) Giammatteo
Dr. Thomas Giammatteo

ANA Publishing
Bloomfield, CT

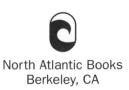

North Atlantic Books
Berkeley, CA

Ex 1: Functional Exercise Program for Women's and Men's Health Issues

Published by
ANA Publishing
800 Cottage Grove Road, Ste. 211
Bloomfield, Connecticut 06002

North Atlantic Books
P.O Box 12327
Berkeley, California 94712

This book is solely educational and informational in nature. The reader of this book agrees that the reader, author, and publisher have not formed a professional, or any other, relationship. The reader assumes full responsibility for any changes or lack of changes experienced due to the reading of this book. The reader also assumes full responsibility for choosing to do any of the activities mentioned in this book. The author and the publisher are not liable for any use or misuse of the information contained herein.

The educational information in this book is not intended for diagnosis, prescription, determination of function, or treatment of any conditions or diseases or any health disorder whatsoever. Readers and students of this method are advised to have a healthcare professional monitor their health. The information in this book should not be used as a replacement for proper medical care.

Any person with disease, pathologies, or accidents should be under the care of a healthcare professional, and consult with them before doing any activity in this book.

Ex 1: Functional Exercise Program for Women's and Men's Health Issues is sponsored by the Society for the Study of Native Arts and Sciences, a nonprofit educational corporation whose goals are to develop an educational and crosscultural perspective linking various scientific, social, and artistic fields; to nurture a holistic view of arts, sciences, humanities, and healing; and to publish and distribute literature on the relationship of mind, body, and nature.

North Atlantic Books' publications are available through most bookstores. For further information, call 800-337-2665 or visit our website at www.northatlanticbooks.com.

Substantial discounts on bulk quantities are available to corporations, professional associations, and other organizations. For details and discount information, contact our special sales department.

Cover and book design by Ayelet Maida, A/M Studios
Photographs by Thomas Giammatteo
Printed in the United States of America

LIBRARY OF CONGRESS CATALOGING-IN-PUBLICATION DATA

(Weiselfish) Giammatteo, Sharon.
    Functional exercise program for women's and men's health issues / developed by Sharon (Weiselfish) Giammatteo; edited by Thomas Giammatteo.
        p. cm. (International College of Integrative Manual Therapy wellness series; 1)
    ISBN 1-55643-366-2 (alk. paper)
    1. Pelvis—Diseases—Exercise therapy.   I. Giammatteo, Thomas.   II. Title.
    III. Series.

RC946 W456 2000
617.5'5062—dc21   00-058235

1 2 3 4 5 6 7 8 9 / 05 04 03 02 01

Contents

Exercise **1**: chair
Exercise **2**: chair
Exercise **3**: chair
Exercise **4**: ice cube, damp washcloth
Exercise **5**: damp washcloth
Exercise **6**: chair, golf ball
Exercise **7**: chair, tennis ball
Exercise **8**: chair, football
Exercise **9**: bed, football
Exercise **10**: bed, tennis ball
Exercise **11**: bed, golf ball
Exercise **12**: chair, golf ball
Exercise **13**: chair, tennis ball
Exercise **14**: chair, football
Exercise **15**: bed, football
Exercise **16**: bed, tennis ball
Exercise **17**: bed, golf ball
Exercise **18**: wall
Exercise **19**: chair, book
Exercise **20**: chair, book
Exercise **21**: toilet
Exercise **22**: toilet
Exercise **23**: toilet
Exercise **24**: toilet
Exercise **25**: toilet
Exercise **26**: toilet
Exercise **27**: toilet
Exercise **28**: toilet
Exercise **29**: bed
Exercise **30**: bed, book

Introduction

The exercises in this book will help all persons, men and women of all ages. With exception to the gender specific exercises in Part 3A and 3B, all the other exercises are meant for both women and men.

The restoration of pelvic function is essential for relief of pain, disease and disability. Persons who suffer from back pain, leg pain, headaches, and spinal disorders may discover that these exercises are useful for decreasing pain and improving function.

Mostly, these exercises are meant for men and women of all ages who tolerate bladder, colon, uterus, cervical, prostate and similar problems. Pain anywhere in the pelvic region can be helped with these exercises. Burning, numbness, tingling and general discomfort of the pelvic floor and lower abdominal region can be helped.

Women who have urinary control problems will be free from stress-incontinence. They will be able to run, skip and jump! They will feel comfortable in different positions which were previously too stressful for bladder control. Sexual activities will be free of the stress of losing bladder control. Pain during menstruation may decrease. Abdominal cramps, constipation and diarrhea will possibly improve. Freedom to participate in sports, leisure activities and work will increase.

Men who fear prostate problems will find that their yearly medical check-ups are good. There will be less discomfort upon urination, and during ejaculation. Men will be able to perform sexual activities with less stress and more ease.

Children who are late bed-wetters may find enormous relief from embarrassment.

These exercises are not meant for single session use. Practice them with all the intentions and motivation expressed in the most important daily rituals. Spend approximately 30 minutes daily for 6 months. After 2 to 3 months the difference will be evident.

There are two approaches to performing these exercises:

1. For mild problems:

Perform these exercises 3 times per week. Spend 30 minutes each session. Use as many exercises as you can fit into the session. Continue with the other exercises during the next session. When you complete all of the exercises, repeat the series. Continue in this manner for 6 months.

2. For significant problems:

Perform these exercises every day. Spend 30 minutes daily. Perform as many exercises as you can fit into the session. Continue with the other exercises the next day, until all of the exercises are performed. Then repeat the series. Continue in this manner for 6 months.

Part **1**

Functional Exercise Program
for Proprioception
of the Pelvic Floor

Exercise **1**

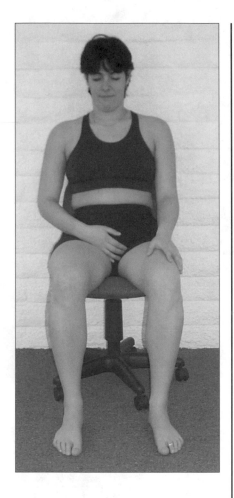

1. Close your eyes.
2. 'Feel' your pelvic region.
3. Touch any part of your pelvic region.
4. Visualize the part you are touching.
5. Open your eyes while you maintain the 'touch.'
6. Change the location of 'touch' each time.

REPETITIONS: 3

SCHEDULE: 3 times a week for 6 months

BENEFIT: This exercise will aid in all pelvic functions.

Exercise **2**

1. Close your eyes.
2. Open your legs to 15 degrees on each side.
3. Open your eyes and look at the 15 degrees abduction (leg opening).
4. Return your legs to midline.
5. Close your eyes.
6. Open your legs to 25 degrees on each side.
7. Open your eyes and look at the 25 degrees abduction (leg opening).
8. Return your legs to midline.
9. Close your eyes.
10. Open your legs to 35 degrees on each side.
11. Open your eyes and look at the 35 degrees abduction (leg opening).
12. Return your legs to midline.

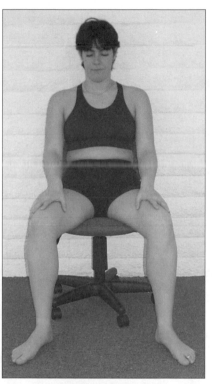

REPETITIONS: 1

SCHEDULE: 3 times a week for 6 months

BENEFIT: This exercise will improve your control of the pelvic region.

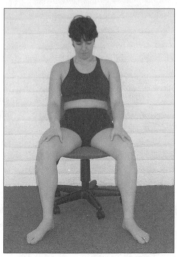

Part **2**

Functional Exercise Program
for Exteroception
of the Pelvic Floor

Exercise **3**

1. Use a 'soft' finger.
2. Touch ALL aspects of the pelvic floor. Cover the entire pelvic area.
3. The touch should be EXTERNAL.
4. Maintain the touch for 2 minutes.

REPETITIONS: 1

SCHEDULE: 3 times a week for 6 months

BENEFIT: This exercise will help decrease pain, numbness, and burning of the pelvic region. It will improve control of all pelvic functions.

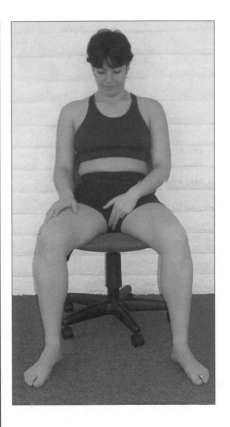

Exercise 4

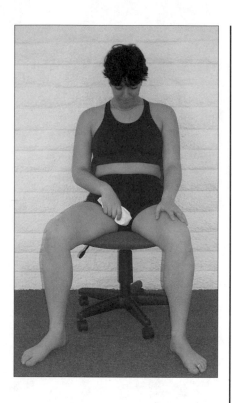

1. Take an ice cube. Wrap the ice cube in a warm, damp wash cloth.
2. Rub the wrapped ice cube GENTLY on all aspects of the pelvic floor. (Best done on bear skin.)
3. The touch should be EXTERNAL.
4. Maintain the touch for 1 minute.

REPETITIONS: 1

SCHEDULE: 3 times a week for 6 months

BENEFIT: This exercise will help decrease pain, numbness, and burning of the pelvic region. The pelvic region will become de-sensitized.

Exercise **5**

1. Take a damp cloth.
2. Place the cloth between your thighs, close to the pelvic floor. (Best done on bear skin.)
3. Pull on the damp cloth while you are closing your legs shut, in order to keep the cloth between your legs. (Isometric resistance)
4. Pull on the cloth with resistance from your thighs for 5 seconds.
5. Relax.

REPETITIONS: 10

SCHEDULE: 3 times a week for 6 months

BENEFIT: This exercise will strengthen the pelvic region. All pelvic functions will improve. This is an excellent exercise for all urinary dribbling and incontinence. Often, women lose urinary control during sexual activities. This exercise will help regain functional control. This is an exercise for severe problems. It is easy to get results.

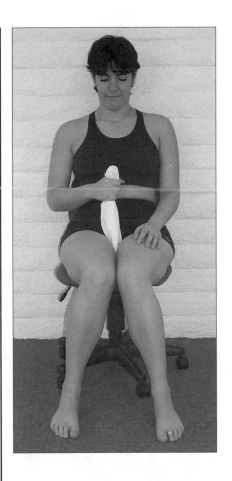

Part **3A**

Functional Exercise Program for Women: Strengthening of the Pelvic Floor

Exercise **6**

1. Place a football between your knees while you are sitting.
2. Squeeze on the football for 1 minute.
3. Relax.

REPETITIONS: 1

SCHEDULE: 3 times a week for 6 months

BENEFIT: This exercise will strengthen the pelvic region. All pelvic functions will improve. This is an excellent exercise for all urinary dribbling and incontinence. Often, women lose urinary control during sexual activities. This exercise will help regain functional control. The upper thighs will be strengthened.

RECOMMENDATION: for mild problems

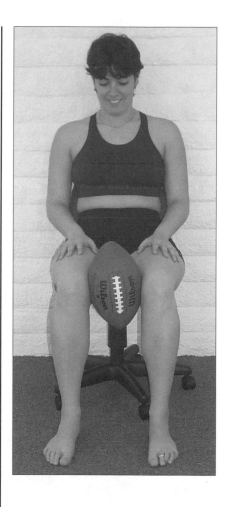

Exercise 7

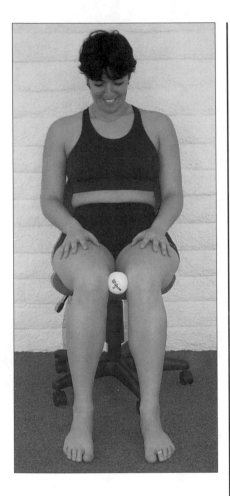

1. Place a tennis ball between your knees while you are sitting.
2. Squeeze on the tennis ball for 1 minute.
3. Relax.

REPETITIONS: 1

SCHEDULE: 3 times a week for 6 months

BENEFIT: This exercise will strengthen the pelvic region. All pelvic functions will improve. This is an excellent exercise for all urinary dribbling and incontinence. Often, women lose urinary control during sexual activities. This exercise will help regain functional control. The upper thighs will be strengthened.

RECOMMENDATION: for mild and moderate problems

Exercise **8**

1. Place a golf ball between your knees while you are sitting.
2. Squeeze on the golf ball for 1 minute.
3. Relax.

REPETITIONSw: 1

SCHEDULE: 3 times a week for 6 months

BENEFIT: This exercise will strengthen the pelvic region. All pelvic functions will improve. This is an excellent exercise for all urinary dribbling and incontinence. Often, women lose urinary control during sexual activities. This exercise will help regain functional control. The upper thighs will be strengthened.

RECOMMENDATION: for moderate and severe problems

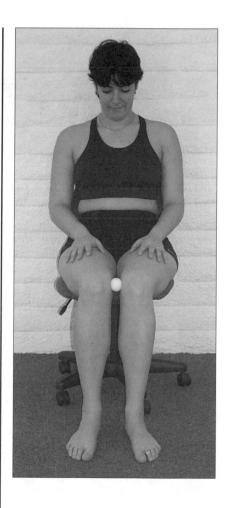

Exercise **9**

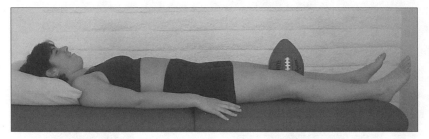

1. Place a football between your knees while you are lying down.
2. Squeeze on the football for 1 minute.
3. Relax.

REPETITIONS: 1

SCHEDULE: 3 times a week for 6 months

BENEFIT: This exercise will strengthen the pelvic region. All pelvic functions will improve. This is an excellent exercise for all urinary dribbling and incontinence. Often, women lose urinary control during sexual activities. This exercise will help regain functional control. The upper thighs will be strengthened.

RECOMMENDATION: for mild problems

Exercise **10**

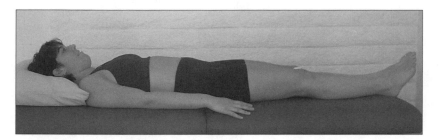

1. Place a tennis ball between your knees while you are lying down.
2. Squeeze on the tennis ball for 1 minute.
3. Relax.

REPETITIONS: 1

SCHEDULE: 3 times a week for 6 months

BENEFIT: This exercise will strengthen the pelvic region. All pelvic functions will improve. This is an excellent exercise for all urinary dribbling and incontinence. Often, women lose urinary control during sexual activities. This exercise will help regain functional control. The upper thighs will be strengthened.

RECOMMENDATION: for moderate and severe problems

Exercise **11**

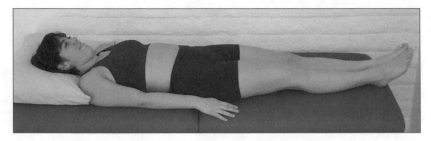

1. Place a golf ball between your knees while you are lying down.
2. Squeeze on the golf ball for 1 minute.
3. Relax.

REPETITIONS: 1

SCHEDULE: 3 times a week for 6 months

BENEFIT: This exercise will strengthen the pelvic region. All pelvic functions will improve. This is an excellent exercise for all urinary dribbling and incontinence. Often, women lose urinary control during sexual activities. This exercise will help regain functional control. The upper thighs will be strengthened.

RECOMMENDATION: for severe problems

Part **3B**

Functional Exercise Program
for Men:
Strengthening
of the Pelvic Floor

Exercise **12**

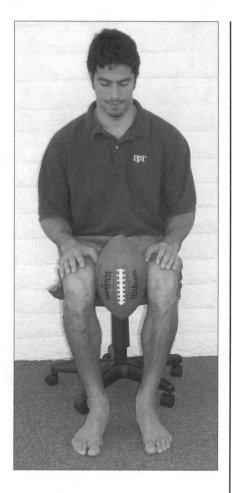

1. Place a football between your knees while you are sitting.
2. Squeeze on the football for 1 minute.
3. Relax.

REPETITIONS: 1

SCHEDULE: 3 times a week for 6 months

BENEFIT: Men have many problems with reflux from the bladder into the prostate. This exercise will help all bladder and prostate problems.

RECOMMENDATION: for mild problems

Exercise **13**

1. Place a tennis ball between your knees while you are sitting.
2. Squeeze on the tennis ball for 1 minute.
3. Relax.

REPETITIONS: 1

SCHEDULE: 3 times a week for 6 months

BENEFIT: Men have many problems with reflux from the bladder into the prostate. This exercise will help all bladder and prostate problems.

RECOMMENDATION: for moderate and severe problems

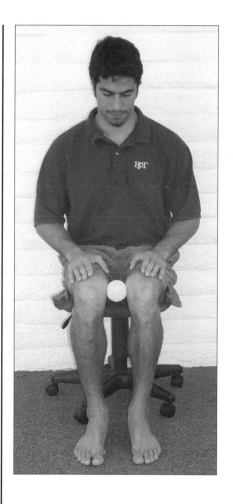

Exercise **14**

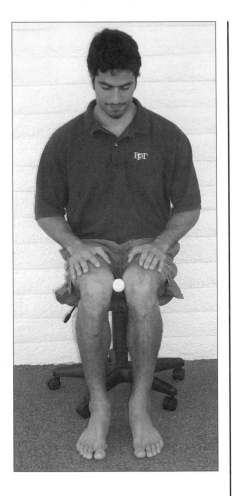

1. Place a golf ball between your knees while you are sitting.
2. Squeeze on the golf ball for 1 minute.
3. Relax.

REPETITIONS: 1

SCHEDULE: 3 times a week for 6 months

BENEFIT: Men have many problems with reflux from the bladder into the prostate. This exercise will help all bladder and prostate problems

RECOMMENDATION: for severe problems

Exercise **15**

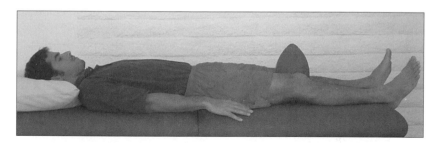

1. Place a football between your knees while you are lying down.
2. Squeeze on the football for 1 minute.
3. Relax.

REPETITIONS: 1

SCHEDULE: 3 times a week for 6 months

BENEFIT: Men have many problems with reflux from the bladder into the prostate. This exercise will help all bladder and prostate problems. This exercise will also help hemorrhoid problems.

RECOMMENDATION: for mild problems

Exercise **16**

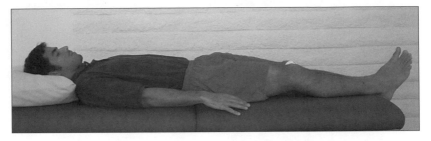

1. Place a tennis ball between your knees while you are lying down.
2. Squeeze on the tennis ball for 1 minute.
3. Relax.

REPETITIONS: 1

SCHEDULE: 3 times a week for 6 months

BENEFIT: Men have many problems with reflux from the bladder into the prostate. This exercise will help all bladder and prostate problems. This exercise will also help hemorrhoid problems.

RECOMMENDATION: for moderate and severe problems

Exercise **17**

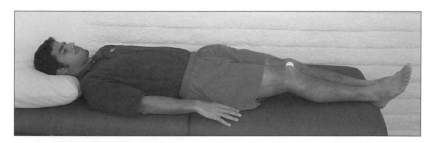

1. Place a golfball between your knees while you are lying down.
2. Squeeze on the golfball for 1 minute.
3. Relax.

REPETITIONS: 1

SCHEDULE: 3 times a week for 6 months

BENEFIT: Men have many problems with reflux from the bladder into the prostate. This exercise will help all bladder and prostate problems. This exercise will also help hemorrhoid problems.

RECOMMENDATION: for severe problems

Exercise **18**

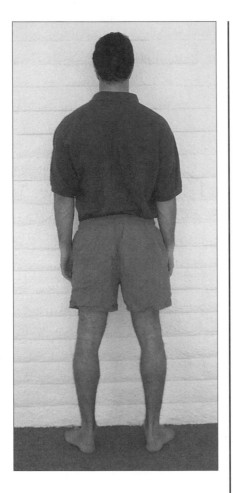

1. Stand up with your face against the wall.
2. Feel the front of your whole body facing the wall.
3. Push your hips forward, against the wall.
4. Maintain this push for 1 minute.

REPETITIONS: 1

SCHEDULE: 3 times a week for 6 months

BENEFIT: This exercise will help low back pain. It is especially helpful for men who have poor urinary flow. It helps restore functional movements for sexual activities.

Exercise **19**

1. Sit on a chair with your feet comfortably resting on the floor.
2. Place a book on your lap.
3. Start to stand up, but do not stand up.

   Do not let the book fall off your lap.

REPETITIONS: 10

SCHEDULE: 3 times a week for 6 months

BENEFIT: This exercise will help low back pain and hip pain. It will help restore sexual function.

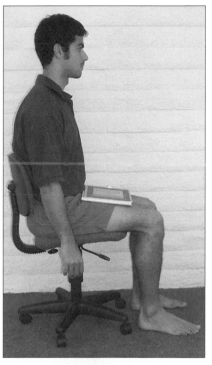

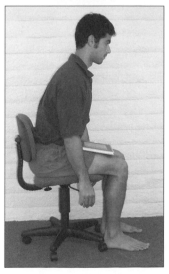

Exercise **20**

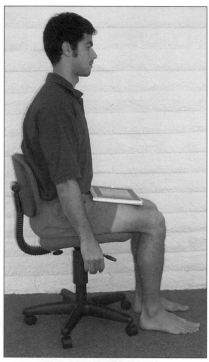

1. Sit on a chair with your feet comfortably resting on the floor.
2. Place a book on your lap.
3. Push both feet into the floor.

   Do not let the book fall off your lap.
4. Maintain the push for 10 seconds.
5. Relax.

REPETITIONS: 3

SCHEDULE: 3 times a week for 6 months

BENEFIT: This exercise will help low back pain, hip pain and leg pain. It will help restore sexual function.

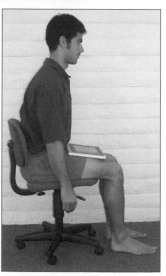

Part **4**

Functional Exercise Program for Re-Education of Urination Function

Exercise **21**

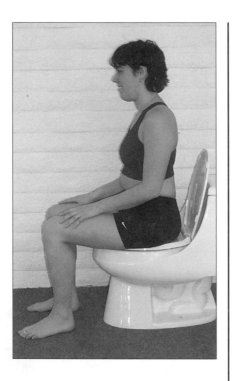

1. When you urinate, stop the flow of urination ONLY ONCE in the middle of the flow.
2. Then continue with the urination process.

REPETITIONS: 1

SCHEDULE: every time you urinate for 6 months

BENEFIT: This exercise will help all bladder function.

RECOMMENDATION: for mild problems

Exercise **22**

When you have urinary frequency:

1. When you urinate, stop the flow of urination TWICE in the middle of the flow.

2. Then continue with the urination process.

REPETITIONS: 1

SCHEDULE: every time you urinate for 6 months

BENEFIT: This exercise will help all bladder function.

RECOMMENDATION: for moderate and severe problems

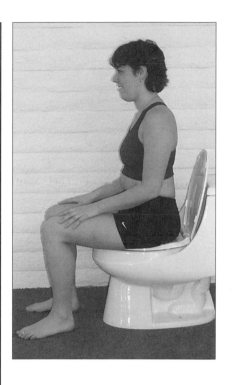

Exercise **23**

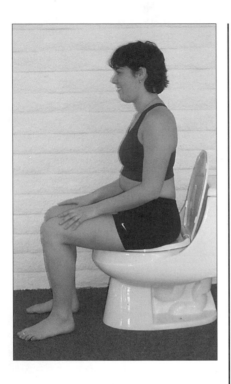

When you have urinary incontinence:

1. When you urinate, stop the flow of urination THREE TIMES in the middle of the flow.
2. Then continue with the urination process.

REPETITIONS: 1

SCHEDULE: every time you urinate for 6 months

BENEFIT: This exercise will help all bladder function. This will be a difficult exercise at the beginning. Within 1 month, the exercise will be easier.

RECOMMENDATION: for severe problems

Exercise **24**

1. Sit on the toilet.
2. Open your legs so that there is a 6 inch distance between your knees.
3. Push your buttocks into the toilet bowl for 10 seconds.
4. Relax.

REPETITIONS: 3

SCHEDULE: 3 times a week for 6 months

BENEFIT: This exercise will help all bladder function. It is good for constipation and diarrhea. It is also good for treatment of hemorrhoid problems. There is usually improvement in low back pain and function.

RECOMMENDATION: for mild, moderate, and severe problems

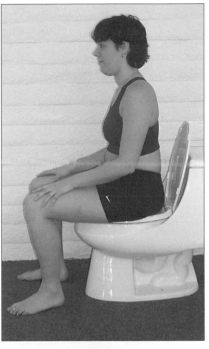

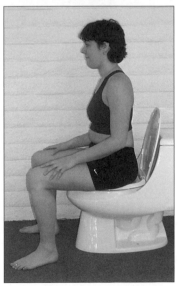

Exercise **25**

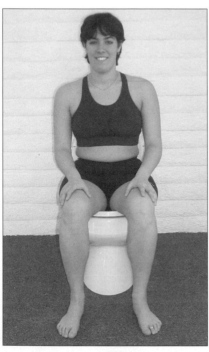

1. Sit on the toilet.
2. Open your legs so that there is a 12 inch distance between your knees.
3. Push your buttocks into the toilet bowl for 10 seconds.
4. Relax.

REPETITIONS: 3

SCHEDULE: 3 times a week for 6 months

BENEFIT: This exercise will help all bladder function. It is good for constipation and diarrhea. It is also good for treatment of hemorrhoid problems. There is usually improvement in low back pain and function.

RECOMMENDATION: for mild, moderate, and severe problems

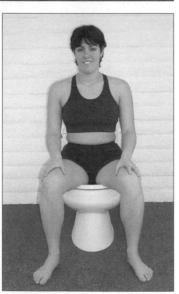

Exercise **26**

1. Sit on the toilet.
2. Cross your legs, so that one knee is on top of the other knee.
3. Push your buttocks into the toilet bowl for 10 seconds.
4. Relax.

REPETITIONS: 3

SCHEDULE: 3 times a week for 6 months

BENEFIT: This exercise will help all bladder function. It is good for constipation and diarrhea. It is also good for treatment of hemorrhoid problems. There is usually improvement in low back, hip pain, and function.

RECOMMENDATION: for mild, moderate, and severe problems

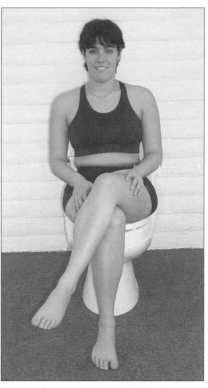

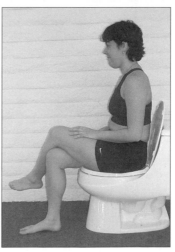

Exercise **27**

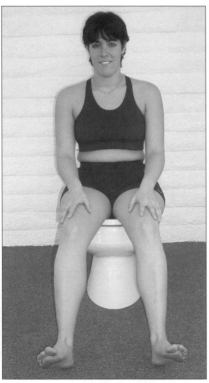

1. Sit on the toilet.
2. Straighten you knees, so that your feet are distant from the toilet bowl.
3. Push your buttocks into the toilet bowl for 10 seconds.
4. Relax.

REPETITIONS: 3

SCHEDULE: 3 times a week for 6 months

BENEFIT: This exercise will help all bladder function. It is good for constipation and diarrhea. It is also good for treatment of hemorrhoid problems. There is usually improvement in low back, hip pain, and function.

RECOMMENDATION: for mild, moderate, and severe problems

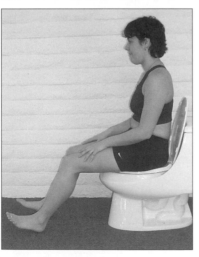

Exercise **28**

1. Sit on the toilet comfortably.
2. Place a book on your lap.
3. Try to stand up, but do not stand up.

   Do not let the book fall from your lap.

4. Relax.

REPETITIONS: 3

SCHEDULE: 3 times a week for 6 months

BENEFIT: This exercise is good for all pelvic functions. Sexual activities are easier with this exercise.

RECOMMENDATION: for mild, moderate, and severe problems

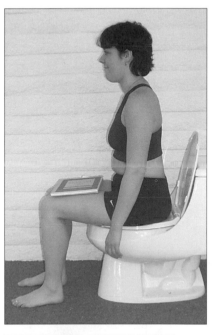

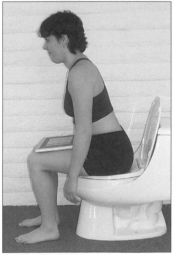

Part **5**

Functional Exercise Program
for Restoration
of Functional Practice

Exercise **29**

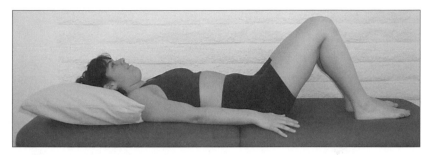

1. Lie on your back on the bed.
2. Bend your hips and knees, so that the soles of your feet are resting on the bed.
3. Push your feet into the bed.
4. Push your buttocks onto the bed.
5. Relax.

REPETITIONS: 3

SCHEDULE: 3 times a week for 6 months

BENEFIT: This exercise is good for all pelvic functions. It improves low back pain and leg weakness. Sexual activities are easier with this exercise.

RECOMMENDATION: for mild. moderate, and severe problems

Exercise **30**

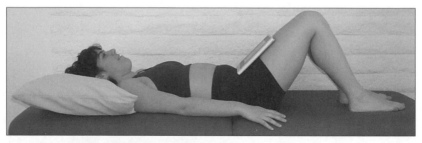

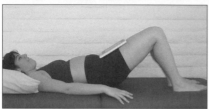

1. Lie on your back on the bed.
2. Bend your hips and knees, so that the soles of your feet are resting on the bed.
3. Place a book on your lap
4. Lift your buttocks off the bed.

   Do not let the book fall off your lap.
5. Relax.

REPETITIONS: 3

SCHEDULE: 3 times a week for 6 months

BENEFIT: This exercise is good for all pelvic functions. It improves low back pain and leg weakness. Sexual activities are easier with this exercise.

RECOMMENDATION: for mild, moderate, and severe problems

Dialogues in Contemporary Rehabilitation

HISTORY OF DIALOGUES IN CONTEMPORARY REHABILITATION

DCR is the company for Integrative Manual Therapy, the Integrated Systems Approach, Integrative Diagnostics, and Functional and Structural Rehabilitation. Founded in the early 1980s by Mary Fiorentino, O.T.,R. Sharon (Weiselfish) Giammatteo initiated a transformation in the educational process incorporated by DCR in 1986, when she received ownership from Mary. Faculty of DCR are trained in all areas of manual therapy; they are experts in the fields of orthopedics and sports medicine, chronic pain, neuro-rehabilitation, pediatrics, geriatrics, women's and men's health issues, cardiopulmonary rehabilitation, and more. Almost 100 percent of the material offered by DCR has been developed, research and present-day results performed, at Regional Physical Therapy in Connecticut.

DCR MISSION STATEMENT

DCR offers hope, practice and purpose. Our goal is recovery; our intention is learning, teaching, and understanding. Our field of accomplishment is extended to client, family, community and world. We accept tomorrow's knowledge as today's quest. We are not hindered by greed, inhibitions, or belief systems. We are multi-denominational, cross-cultural, and non-racial in orientation. We wish to facilitate recovery from dysfunction through growth and development.

Biomechanics with: Muscle Energy and 'Beyond' Technique
MET1: Pelvis, Sacrum and Spine
MET2: Upper and Lower Extremities and Rib Cage
MET3: Advanced Biomechanics: Sacrum and Spine
MET4: Type III Biomechanical Dysfunction: Spine and Extremities and Bone Bruises

Muscle and Circulation with Strain and Counterstrain Technique
SCS1: Strain and Counterstrain for Orthopedics and Neurologic Patient
SCS2: Advanced Strain and Counterstrain for Autonomic Nervous System

Connective Tissue with Myofascial Release, The 3-Planar Fascial Fulcrum Technique
MFR1: Myofascial Release for Orthopedic, Neurologic, Geriatric Patient
MFR2: Myofascial Mapping for Integrative Diagnostics

Peripheral Nerve Tissue Tension: Hypomobility and Fibrosis
NTT2: Neural Tissue Tension Technique

Cranial and the Craniosacral System with: The Cranial Therapy Series
CTS1: Osseous, Suture, Joint and Membrane
CTS2: Membrane, Fluid, Facial Vault and Cranial Gear-Complex
CTS3: Cranial Diaphragm Compression Syndromes; CSF Fluid: Production, Distribution and Absorption; Immunology
CTS4: Neuronal Regeneration, Cranial Nerves, and Neurotransmission
CTSA1: Postural Reflexes
CTSA2: Vasculature in the Brain
CTSA3: The Eye

Organs with Visceral Mobilization
VMET1: Visceral Mobilization with Muscle Energy and 'Beyond'— Focus GI Tract
VMET2: Women's and Men's Health Issues
VMET3: Respiratory Rehabilitation
VMET4: Cardiac Habilitation
VMET5: The Liver

The Lymphatic System
LYM1: Congestion Therapy
LYM2: Immune Preference

Compression Syndromes
COMP1: Compression Syndromes of the Upper Extremities
COMP2: Compression Syndromes of the Lower Extremities
COMP3: Diaphragm Compression Syndromes

Neuro-Rehabilitation
DMT: Developmental Manual Therapy for the Neurologic Patient

Integrative Diagnostics
IDS: Integrative Diagnostic Series: Myofascial Mapping,
Neurofascial Process, Rx Plans
IDAP: Integrative Diagnostics for Applied Psychosynthesis
IDLB: Integrative Diagnostics for Lower Back

Integrative Seminars
IMTS: Integrative Manual Therapy for Neck, Thoracic Outlet,
Shoulder and Upper Extremity
IMTUE/LESM: Integrative Manual Therapy for Upper and Lower
Extremities in Sports Medicine
IMTCCC: Integrative Manual Therapy for Craniocervical,
Craniofacial, Craniomandibular

Functional Rehabilitation
Therapeutic Horizons: The Brain (BANM); The Heart (BACM);
The Pelvis (BANRA); Advanced Levels 1–3 (BAAL1–3)

NES & DCR Offer Adjunct Educational Material
in Integrative Manual Therapy

BOOKS

Manual Therapy for the Pelvis, Sacrum, Cervical, Thoracic and Lumbar Spine, with Muscle Energy Technique—A Contemporary Clinical Analysis of Biomechanics by Sharon Weiselfish, Ph.D., P.T.

Integrative Manual Therapy for the Autonomic Nervous System and Related Disorders by Thomas Giammatteo, D.C. P.T., and Sharon (Weiselfish) Giammatteo, Ph.D., P.T.

Integrative Manual Therapy for the Upper and Lower Extremities, Introducing Synergic Pattern Release with Strain and Counterstrain Technique, and Muscle Energy and 'Beyond' Technique for the Peripheral Joints by Sharon (Weiselfish) Giammatteo, Ph.D., P.T., edited by Thomas Giammatteo, D.C., P.T.

By Sharon (Weiselfish) Giammatteo, Ph.D., P.T.
Produced by Northeast Seminars

Muscle Energy Technique Series
  #1 Pelvis
  #2 Sacrum
  #3 Thoracic and Lumbar Spine
  #4 Cervical and Thoracic Spine
  #5 Strain and Counterstrain for the Orthopedic and Neurologic
    Patient
  #6 Myofascial Release, the 3-Planar Fascial Fulcrum Approach,
    for the Orthopedic, Neurologic and Geriatric Patient
  #7 Advanced Manual Therapy for the Low Back
  #8 Integrative Manual Therapy: A Patient in Process
  #9 Manual Therapy for the Low Back: Standards for the Health
    Care Industry for the 21st Century
 #10 Muscle Energy and 'Beyond' Technique for the Upper
    Extremities
 #11 Muscle Energy and 'Beyond' Technique for the Lower
    Extremities

For further information regarding educational products,
please contact Northeast Seminars at:

Northeast Seminars
P.O. Box 522
East Hampstead, NH 03826
Tel: 800-272-2044
Fax: 603-329-7045
E-mail: neseminar@aol.com
Website: www.neseminars.com

For further information regarding DCR products and seminars,
please contact DCR at:

DCR
Dialogues in Contemporary Rehabilitation
800 Cottage Grove Road, Suite 211
Bloomfield, CT 06002
Tel: 860-243-5220
Fax: 860-243-5304
E-mail: dcrhealth@aol.com
Website: www.dcrhealth.com

Exercise Program

PATIENT NAME _____ **DATE** _____

HEALTHCARE PRACTITIONER _____ **PHONE** _____

6 MONTH SESSION BEGINS _____

SESSION FREQUENCY: ☐ Daily ☐ 3 times a week

Perform the following exercises for 30 minutes per session.
Follow specific instructions for each exercise.

☐ Exercise **1**	☐ Exercise **11**	☐ Exercise **21**
☐ Exercise **2**	☐ Exercise **12**	☐ Exercise **22**
☐ Exercise **3**	☐ Exercise **13**	☐ Exercise **23**
☐ Exercise **4**	☐ Exercise **14**	☐ Exercise **24**
☐ Exercise **5**	☐ Exercise **15**	☐ Exercise **25**
☐ Exercise **6**	☐ Exercise **16**	☐ Exercise **26**
☐ Exercise **7**	☐ Exercise **17**	☐ Exercise **27**
☐ Exercise **8**	☐ Exercise **18**	☐ Exercise **28**
☐ Exercise **9**	☐ Exercise **19**	☐ Exercise **29**
☐ Exercise **10**	☐ Exercise **20**	☐ Exercise **30**

Notes

Exercise Program

Perform the following exercises for 30 minutes per session.
Follow specific instructions for each exercise.

☐ Exercise **1**	☐ Exercise **11**	☐ Exercise **21**
☐ Exercise **2**	☐ Exercise **12**	☐ Exercise **22**
☐ Exercise **3**	☐ Exercise **13**	☐ Exercise **23**
☐ Exercise **4**	☐ Exercise **14**	☐ Exercise **24**
☐ Exercise **5**	☐ Exercise **15**	☐ Exercise **25**
☐ Exercise **6**	☐ Exercise **16**	☐ Exercise **26**
☐ Exercise **7**	☐ Exercise **17**	☐ Exercise **27**
☐ Exercise **8**	☐ Exercise **18**	☐ Exercise **28**
☐ Exercise **9**	☐ Exercise **19**	☐ Exercise **29**
☐ Exercise **10**	☐ Exercise **20**	☐ Exercise **30**

Notes

Exercise Program

PATIENT NAME _____ **DATE** _____

HEALTHCARE PRACTITIONER _____ **PHONE** _____

6 MONTH SESSION BEGINS _____

SESSION FREQUENCY: ☐ Daily ☐ 3 times a week

Perform the following exercises for 30 minutes per session.
Follow specific instructions for each exercise.

☐ Exercise **1**	☐ Exercise **11**	☐ Exercise **21**
☐ Exercise **2**	☐ Exercise **12**	☐ Exercise **22**
☐ Exercise **3**	☐ Exercise **13**	☐ Exercise **23**
☐ Exercise **4**	☐ Exercise **14**	☐ Exercise **24**
☐ Exercise **5**	☐ Exercise **15**	☐ Exercise **25**
☐ Exercise **6**	☐ Exercise **16**	☐ Exercise **26**
☐ Exercise **7**	☐ Exercise **17**	☐ Exercise **27**
☐ Exercise **8**	☐ Exercise **18**	☐ Exercise **28**
☐ Exercise **9**	☐ Exercise **19**	☐ Exercise **29**
☐ Exercise **10**	☐ Exercise **20**	☐ Exercise **30**

Notes